Your Best Body Now!

Real Advice from 10 Top Trainers

United Print Publishers

DEDICATION

This book is dedicated to all of the incredible professionals and companies who took the time to submit content to this book. It has been a pleasure working with each of you, on the production of this book. The time you have all taken and the high quality content that you have all shared has truly gone above and beyond anything we could have ever expected when we first set out to publish this book. Thank you to everyone who made this possible.

UNITED PRINT PUBLISHERS

DISCLAIMER

This book is an educational product that provides general health information. The materials In "YOUR BEST BODY NOW!: REAL ADVICE FROM 10 TOP TRAINERS" are provided "as is" and without warranties of any kind either express or implied.

AS AN EXPRESS CONDITION TO USING THE INFORMATION IN THIS BOOK, YOU MUST AGREE TO THE FOLLOWING TERMS. IF YOU DISAGREE WITH ANY OF THESE TERMS, DO NOT USE THE INFORMATION IN THIS BOOK. YOUR PARTICIPATION IN ACTIVITIES MENTIONED IN THIS BOOK MEANS THAT YOU ARE AGREEING TO BE LEGALLY BOUND BY THESE TERMS:

This book's content is not a substitute for direct, personal, professional medical care and diagnosis. None of the advice, diet plans, or exercises mentioned should be performed or otherwise used without clearance from your physician or health care provider. The information contained within is not intended to provide specific physical or mental health advice, or any other advice whatsoever, for any individual or company and should not be relied upon in that regard. We are not medical professionals and nothing in this book should be misconstrued to mean otherwise.

There may be risks associated with participating in activities mentioned in this book, for people in poor health or with pre-existing physical or mental health conditions. Because these risks exist, you should not participate in such diet plans if you are in poor health or have a pre-existing mental or physical condition. If you choose to follow any advice within this book, you do so of your own free will and accord, knowingly and voluntarily assuming all risks associated with such activities.

Facts and information are believed to be accurate at the time they were published in this book. All information provided is to be used for informational purposes only. Products and services described are only offered in jurisdictions where they may be legally offered. Information provided is not all-inclusive, and is limited to information that is made available. Such information should not be relied upon as all-inclusive or accurate.

You agree to hold UNITED PRINT PUBLISHERS, its owners, agents, and employees harmless from any and all liability for all claims for damages due to injuries, including attorney fees and costs, incurred by you or caused to third parties by you, arising out of the fitness and diet plans discussed in this book.

Testimonials, case studies, and examples within this book are unverified results that have been forwarded to us by the interviewees featured in this book, and may not reflect the typical reader's experience, may not apply to the average person, and are not intended to represent or guarantee that anyone will achieve the same or similar results. You should always perform due diligence and not take such results at face value. We are not responsible for any errors or omissions in typical results information supplied to us by third parties.

CONTENTS

ACKNOWLEDGMENTS

Epic Evolution Fitness, LLC.
Healthy Now, Healthy For Life, LLC
Fitness Integration Training – F.I.T
Indianapolis Fitness and Sports Training
Life Fitness Academy
Barry's Bootcamp
Steps Inc.
American Mobile Fitness
Studio Element
Center-Fit

Thank you to the following fitness experts who without their contributions and support this book would not have been written: Ava Ford, Robert Lekan, Matthew Webster, Lance Goyke, Terry Barga, Derrick Sobotka, Irv Rubenstein, Gregg Schwartz, Jay Siefert, and Steve & Tori Bradford.

INTRODUCTION

If you've ever spent any amount of time strolling through the "Fitness & Nutrition" books section, at your local book store, you've probably noticed one thing: There sure are a lot of books on the subject of losing weight and eating healthy. While this large amount of information on the subject may seem like a good thing, it could also be the one thing that keeps you from taking action towards your personal fitness and nutrition goals.

As you're probably aware, the fitness and nutrition industry is a multi-billion dollar industry. There are thousands upon thousands of people who rely on you to buy the next fitness book, exercise gadget, or DVD that hits the store shelves or the late night TV airwaves. Unfortunately, in this profit-driven world known as the fitness and nutrition industry, one priority gets lost: Getting real results for the end-user. You see, if one of these multi-million dollar companies actually produced a gadget or DVD that enabled everyone to be in the best shape of their lives forever, you wouldn't need to buy their products anymore - and that's exactly what they don't want to happen!

So what does this mean for you? Should you just throw in the towel and give up on any and all information out there? Of course not. You do, however, need to be more selective in where you get your information from.

The goal of this book was to interview real personal trainers who really train clients each and every day of their professional lives. When we produced this book, we set out to find real world experts and that's exactly what we got. Our biggest challenge was getting these personal trainers to break away from their busy schedules of training their clients, so that they could actually share their advice in this book. The trainers who have contributed to this book "walk the walk", and the content they've provided, in the following chapters, reflects their true knowledge and expertise. So, without further ado, we present to you, the real world expert interviews!

INTERVIEW WITH AVA FORD

1 SUCCEEDING MENTALLY FIRST

Epic Evolution Fitness specializes in personalized fitness programming, group sessions, and corporate wellness. Specialty areas include performance enhancement, corrective exercise, flexibility and mobility and myofascial release.

Is it better to exercise every part of the body on the same day, or is it better to focus on different muscle groups on different days? Please explain why one is better than the other.

I lean toward total body training for all of my clients. The movements experienced in everyday living require the recruitment of several muscle groups so training in this fashion results in improved movement quality and efficiency and safe execution of these movement patterns as well. Functional movement programs typically include 2-3 days of resistance training. Isolating muscle groups can be beneficial as well depending on the individual goals. For example, someone that is striving to gain more upper body strength may choose to have a day that is more heavily loaded with upper body exercises.

Should women lift weights if they don't want to get bulky looking? If yes, how can they lift weights and not get that bulky/masculine look?

ALL women should lift weights. While they are built differently and genetics play a large role in muscle fiber type and distribution, females do not have the natural ability to develop the large mass that men do. Resistance training actually leads to higher calorie burn throughout the workout as well as calorie burning afterward during EPOC (Excess Post Oxygen Consumption) while the body is returning to homeostasis. This being said, the inclusion of weight training leads to increased calorie and fat burning, weight loss, increased muscle strength and eventually definition.

Is it true that some people naturally lose weight faster than others? Why or why not is this the case?

Genetics and metabolism do allow some individuals to lose or maintain a healthy weight more so than others. However, several other factors impact successful weight loss. Factors include amount of sleep, stress level, rate of metabolism, exercise frequency and duration, drinking, medications, stress level, and diagnosed or undiagnosed diseases and conditions.

What precautions should seniors take into consideration, when starting a new exercise program?

Older active adults and anyone looking to start a new training program should consult a physician first. Conditions such as osteoporosis, cardiovascular disease, high blood pressure, cancer and diabetes to name a few, need to be identified beforehand in order for a safe and effective personalized training program to be created.

Is it typical for a personal trainer to ask their clients to sign a contract? If so, what are some standard contract lengths and terms?

An individual that is participating in personalized training needs to be involved in some sort of program in order to form healthy habits that are conducive to achieving goals. Inconsistently scheduled sessions are not going to produce the desired results. Most clients need at least 6 weeks to see true results. While contract lengths vary, a 6 month to 1 year program would yield the best, most concrete results.

If someone enjoys drinking alcohol in moderation, how often can they indulge without feeling guilty or undoing all the progress they made with their trainer?

Alcohol can be ok as long as it is done in moderation. One drink 2-3 times a week won't wreck an individual's fitness goals as long as calorie count and sugar are kept in mind. Some alcohols, such as red wine offer heart health benefits when enjoyed with discretion. Think about it this way, do you want to eat your calories or drink them? The body is an amazing machine. It is pushed to it's limits during training and deserves to be treated healthfully. This is important to remember when making nutritional and lifestyle decisions.

What can people do if they "plateau" and stop seeing results from their workout routine?

When an individual reaches a plateau, their body is no longer experiencing increases in neural demands and little to no improvements are experienced.

Manipulating acute training variables once this point is reached results in increased demands being placed on the central nervous system. Acute variables include repetitions, sets, intensity, tempo, rest intervals, frequency, duration, and exercise selection.

Is it true that genetics or body physiology make it impossible for some people to get in shape?

Genetics determine the amount of muscle mass we are able to gain naturally and performance abilities. They do not limit anyone from getting into shape unless the individual is experiencing a thyroid or mobility issue. If you can move, you can work toward a better, stronger, healthier version of yourself. Fitness journeys require hard work, discipline, and adherence. Remember, it is never too late to be in the best shape of your life, you have to want it and work for it.

What is the "fat burning zone" that trainers often refer to?

The oxidative energy system, which is utilized during sustain low to moderate exercise, is the metabolic system that uses triglycerides in the presence of oxygen for the production of ATP, our energy source. When exercise is performed at about 45-70% aerobic capacity, this the main energy system used to sustain exercise.

Do people really lose muscle as they get older? If so, how much muscle do they lose on average, and can anything be done to slow down this process?

Aging results in degenerative processes including decreased neural proprioception, depleted strength, endurance, and overall muscle mass. Physical inactivity results in about a 5% loss in muscle mass after the age of 30. The good news is that these processes can be slowed by engaging in regular physical activity to include both resistance training and cardiovascular conditioning.

Is it safe to workout first thing in the morning, on an empty stomach?

Breakfast is essential in terms of weight loss and overall performance. Even if you find that you do not have an appetite upon waking, it is still good practice to feed your body. Waiting too long to eat, at any time of day, causes the body to store calories. Eating a small meal, such as a protein shake or bar, and a piece of fruit helps regulate blood glucose and jump start metabolic processes which decreases the chances of cravings which could lead to poor nutritional choices.

Is it true that it's good to have a "cheat day" where people can eat whatever they want once a week? Why is this a good or bad idea?

The impact of nutrition on exercise performance is important to consider. Many individuals treat themselves to a "cheat day" for maintaining good fitness and nutritional habits throughout the week. While there is nothing wrong with this practice, overindulging in excess calories, fat, and other "junk" may negatively impact performance and increase the amount of time taken to reach SMART (Specific, Measurable, Attainable, Realistic, Timely) fitness goals. Mindfulness is key. It is ok to treat yourself every once in a while as long as portion size and nutritional value are kept in mind. While I wouldn't recommend a full day of poor nutritional choices, maybe opt for one meal or a couple snacks throughout one day. For example, if you have a craving for pizza, look up a healthy recipe. That way you can enjoy the food, monitor the quality of the food being consumed and also know that your nutritional habits aren't taking a big hit!

HOW TO CONTACT US

Ava Ford

Founder and CEO of Epic Evolution Fitness, LLC.

Website: www.e2fitnessllc.com

Email: e2fitness@outlook.com

Phone: 214-335-6240

2 HOW TO LIVE A HEALTHY LIFESTYLE

The emphasis is on balance, integrated and holistic viewpoint of health and wellness. Health is not meant to be just physical, but through mental and emotional wellbeing by employing a network of trained and certified practitioners of various modalities to help the client reach their ultimate state of wellbeing.

If someone eats very healthy, and they have an active lifestyle, do they still need to workout? Why or why not?

They do need to work out for several reasons. Working out not only helps being physically healthy, it helps with movement, daily living as well as helping their mental and emotional states. When a person works out, they are able to handle better higher levels of stress without detriment to their own health. They are able to help move through their body in a pain free state.

As many people today deal with issues of being in a sitting, lethargic and cramped work environment, the mental and sometimes emotional stress they encounter at their job forces their body to tighten and stiffen, causing imbalances and physical issues. Pain inhibits movement. Lack of movement or improper movement causes a person to remain more in a stationary state. Lack of activity wears on the mental and emotional well-being on a person helping to cause them to create situations, (poor eating habits, depression, etc), further spiraling them in to an unhealthy situation. Working out is one part, but an easier part for a client to do for themselves by themselves.

How can a personal trainer help a client, with regard to nutrition?

A well informed trainer often meets with a client more often than a doctor or most other health professional. A well informed trainer can help talk with a client, monitor their eating habits, track their results more often and be able to give them feedback and better direction more immediately then most health professionals which are seen perhaps once to twice a month or even year.

What are some examples of foods that people think are good for them, but they're really not, and why are these foods actually not healthy?

Most people focus on low fat foods, especially when they are prepackaged and prepared foods. Salad dressings, cookies and other foods trick most people in to thinking they are eating something they enjoy without doing much harm to their actual bodies. Most that are low fat are replaced with chemicals or sugars to mimic the flavors they crave, which doesn't create a better health, just shifts the unhealthy calories and intake in another direction, such as being addicted to diet drinks, sugar or other substances.

What are some factors that impact people's metabolism?

Blood sugar and the lack awareness of what people eat. Most people are unaware of what they eat and why they are eating them. The cycle that tends to be seen is when they feel low, depressed or having a bad day they tend to mindlessly eat. When that happens, they tend to over eat, snack on packaged food filled with sugar or poly saturated fat which makes them feel better and also spikes their blood sugar.

This produces a temporary high if good feelings and spikes the blood sugar. When the blood sugar spikes, the body produces insulin to help deal with the intake of sugar. When the sugar intake in consistently too high, as tends to happen with a processed carb heavy diet, the body can't produce enough insulin to deal with it and it becomes insulin resistant. This adds to a higher fat in the body, slower metabolism and predispositions people to become pre-diabetic or diabetic. Also more people tend to pay attention to the bigger words or not taking the time to understand labels on food, causing them not be able to understand what is and what isn't healthy.

Is there any true benefit to warming up, cooling down, or stretching before or after exercising? If there is, why are these things important?

There are benefits for all of them. Warming up not only increases your range of motion, prepares your body for a workout by not only increasing your blood flow but with increasing the sensory systems of your body. It also helps to activate your mind and puts it on alert to be aware of how you are using your body and to be aware of how it feels when working out. This does not mean normal static stretching of just holding a stretch through a held position, this is more in terms of dynamic stretching and allowing the body to move through a motion.

Cooling down and stretching I tend to put in the same. This does not mean they are the same. Cooling down can mean breathing techniques, stretching, ice baths and so on. This allows the body to begin the repair stage and rejuvenation of the body. It allows the heart rate to slow down and for any muscles/joints that need to prepare to be opened can at that time.

Once someone begins working out with a personal trainer, what goes on during the sessions?

That is pretty much up to the client and the trainer. Every trainer has his or her formula that works for them and what they perceive with their client. Warming up, dynamic stretching, stabilization exercises, balance, core, strength, cardio, plyometrics, boxing, tai chi, Qi gong etc... Every trainer has their method. What should typically happens is a greeting, some short induction on how the client is feeling, any issues they have going on, a quick review of what of a plan for during the session, the actual session and possibly some sort of cool down if there is time or if the client requests it.

How can people accurately determine how many calories they burn during a workout?

The best way these days is a calorie counter. Several companies have them, many with a heart rate monitor with an estimated calories burned. This varies per model. It will give a good ratio or idea, but exact counts can be hard to figure out. The ones given on a cardio machine are rarely accurate, the best for a personal count is something that you wear throughout a workout and has some personal information about your body.

What should someone look for in a good health club/gym?

What should be decided before someone ever looks at a health club is to decide what they need it for. If it is mainly to do cardio and maybe some crunches, minimal equipment should be looked for. If it is something more specific or the client needs a variety, making sure there is a wide variety of options or goes in the vein of what the specific goals and needs are. What should be looked for is a clean gym, functioning equipment, friendly staff. Make sure all areas are looked at and you feel comfortable with it all.

How can people prevent joint injuries or sore joints when lifting weights?

First of all, start slowly. If you haven't been to a gym from a few months to never, you should start slowly. Your body can't go from 0 to 100 in a 6 seconds, it needs to be warmed up. If you are unsure about things, this would be a good time to start with a trainer to understand basics with form, understand with how stable they are in their body and a general course of action.

If your body is out of alignment it will not function correctly. If you add weight and speed to a dysfunctioning body, you will just exasperate the issues and make them worse. Making sure you move correctly is the first step, then moving correctly consistently is the next.

What types of scheduling commitments are customary, when hiring a personal trainer? In other words, do people normally take things one week at a time or are they typically asked to schedule several weeks at a time with their trainer?

Every trainer is different as each client. It is typical to schedule week by week, with sometime during the previous week the next week's session/s will be decided. Some clients who are about to have a crazy hectic week will want to schedule a few weeks in advanced, but that is up to the client and what they need.

What if someone is completely out of shape? What's the safest approach for getting started?

Slowly. Many clients like to jump in to the thick of things and start off hard core, which tends to be the biggest mistake. Start slowly but consistently. Make sure workouts are planned and kept. Even if it is 45 minutes of walking on a treadmill, it is a start. The biggest thing is to move slowly and consistently, if you stumble one day, then make sure you start again the next day and not to try and double your efforts.

Add changes slowly, one or two per every two to three weeks. They are supposed to be meaningful changes, they won't happen overnight. And that is the other thing, to be safe, you have to be patient. Every client can make their goal, but if they don't understand that this is a slow process and it won't happen overnight, then they will easily get frustrated or they will try and push themselves way beyond their limit, feel like they are failing and quit. Keep things in perspective and look at the big picture. It will happen.

HOW TO CONTACT US

Rob Lekan

Owner of Healthy Now, Healthy For Life, LLC

PersonalTrainerRobChi@gmail.com

3 TIPS FOR BEST RESULTS

My business provides at-home and on-site personal training services. It's all about providing a convenient service for individuals or groups looking to get F.I.T in the comfort of their own home or place of work.

What are the best types of exercises for getting the fastest results in the shortest period of time?

Compound exercises will get the fastest results. An example is a Squat Thruster – a squat with dumbbell shoulder press. The more muscles you work with each exercise the more energy your body will have to produce to perform the exercise.

Is it true that people with diabetes have a harder time losing weight? If so, why is this the case?

It's very important that individuals with diabetes discuss exercise with their doctors. Weight loss can be achieved by both type 1 & 2 diabetics. It may be harder for people with diabetes to lose weight initially until a fitness routine becomes consistent and (1) frequently check blood glucose levels, (2) learn what type of fast acting carbohydrates work best in case of a hypoglycemic episode, (3) figure out the best time of day to exercise each day, (4) how to snack before and during exercise, (5) and get all these variables in order with their doctors.

If someone hasn't worked out in years, how should they get started in the safest way possible?

It would be good to start by meeting with a personal trainer to discussing exercise history and health history. Then create a workout program which includes cardio and strength training. Two key factors when starting a program is to learn good lifting form and to build into your program. Don't start off too quick or the high levels of soreness or injury will keep you from being consistent.

What are some of the most common myths about building muscle?

A popular myth is that you have to lift heavy weights to build muscles. Muscles strength is determined by the amount of stress put on it while lifting. Light weight and high reps builds muscles and is less stressful on the joint.

Do people need exercise equipment to get in shape?

You don't need exercise equipment to get in shape. There are lots of body weight exercises that can be performed in any space, such as squats, pushups, variations of situps, and yoga poses to name a few. If you can't go outside to run, bike, or walk, there are other forms of cardio that don't require much space, such as jumping jacks, high knees, butt kicks... With a little research you'd be amazed by how many at-home workouts you can find that don't require any equipment.

Is weight lifting a good idea for people who have high blood pressure?

Weight lifting should supplement cardio training. It's important the individuals don't hold their breath or overly strain while lifting and isometric exercises should be avoided. Weight lifting should incorporate low resistance and higher number of repetitions.

Is it dangerous to take supplements?

Supplements can be dangerous. There's a chance of overdose, unnecessary strain on the organs trying to digest them and can be very expensive. Most healthy adults will get the same results with diet consisting of veggies, fruits, and lean meats. Always talk to your doctor before adding a supplement to your daily plan.

Does it make a difference if someone just does all of their exercise over the weekend as compared to spreading it out over the week?

Working out on the weekends is a good start to a fitness program. It's recommended that people get moderate activity almost daily. Depending on your fitness level it would be best to workout 3-5 times per week, but also be as active as possible through each day by standing up and walking around as much as possible.

Is coffee bad for someone who's trying to lose weight or get in shape?

Most things are good in moderation. Coffee can be a way for someone to curb a carving by drinking their snack instead of hitting up the vending machine. A lot of people drink coffee before they workout for an energy increase. If you have any health issues make sure to discuss coffee drinking before a workout with your doctor. Overall, coffee can benefit weight loss and getting in shape.

Is aerobic walking as healthy as jogging or running?

This all depends on the individual's fitness level. If you are a beginner or someone with foot, ankle, knee, or hips issues walking is a very healthy option. If your goal is to advance your fitness level then jogging and running will be a more efficient option.

Can someone still lose weight if they split their workouts throughout the day?

It's important to accumulate at least 30 minutes of activity daily. This can be done all at once or broken down into intervals. Either way you are boosting your metabolism and your carbs 'out' will increase and weight loss can be the result.

What are the must-have items that someone should bring with them to a personal training session?

Individuals should bring water for hydration and a towel to wipe off the sweat! Everything else will most likely be provided for by the trainer.

HOW TO CONTACT US

Matthew Webster

Owner of Fitness Integration Training – F.I.T

Email: mwebsfitness@gmail.com

Website: www.fitnessintegrationtraining.com

Phone: 402-525-1744

4 PREPARING FOR YOUR WORKOUT

IFAST is a world-known place where people come to get fixed. It's difficult to capture in words, but we're the trainers that other trainers refer out to. LanceGoyke.com is my private affiliate where I offer distance coaching in addition to free blog material.

What is the correct way to breathe when working out?

The way you breathe when working out is entirely dependent on what kind of exercise you're doing.

First, there's exercise that taxes the cardiorespiratory system. This kind of exercise requires you to breathe a lot more than your normal activities, so you're expected to take more and quicker breaths. You notice this a lot with exercises that are generally called "cardio" - e.g. running, rowing, swimming.

If I'm exercising with lighter weights in a circuit fashion, I generally want an inhale during the "stretching" part of the movement and an exhale during the "hard" part of the movement. Take a squat for example - inhale on the way down, exhale on the way up. If I've given someone an extra slow exercise that is developing how your muscles use the oxygen they receive, then I'll just cue the client to maintain their breathing.

If I'm doing heavy strength training, however, I don't want any breathing! Subtle movements occur at the spine and rib cage when you breathe in and out, but you don't want to deal with those when you're under a lot of load. Hold your breath throughout the movement to protect your spine.

When you're about to lift something heavy, follow this three step process:

(1) Set your ribs down towards your hips with a full exhale - "full" meaning "blowing out all the candles on your 106th birthday cake".

(2) Make yourself feel really "tall".

(3) Take a big breath into your back.

One more scenario is for the client who has recurring pains throughout their body. As a coach, I may not be able to see all the little nuances going on inside you with my eyes.

What I do in this case is make you hold the most difficult position of an exercise, and then take a breath. If the breath looks good, then you're in the right position. I'll use this when I'm working out to "coach" myself - if the breath feels right, I'm in the right position.

But what does a good breath look like?

B

Film yourself taking a deep breath to see what part of your body is moving when you take your air in. You want your whole torso to fill at the same time - air expanding the chest and belly out to the front, back, and sides. The most common mistake is not filling up the backside of the body during an inhale. Instead, the air is pulled in by the neck and the belly gets skinnier. On an exhale, you want the reverse to happen. You'll need a strong midsection to get air out AND to get air in the right way.

Now watch your video again and look at your face. If it looks strained, you're doing it wrong.

E

The most widespread problem is that almost everyone, much like Whitney Houston, is waiting to exhale, but never does. If I had only two words to explain proper breathing, they would be "exhale more". A full exhale sets you up for a better inhale and helps you relax.

N

You'll generally want to breathe in your nose and out your mouth. If you find yourself hyperventilating a lot, use only your nose.

D

Fewer, deep breaths are preferred over more, shallow breaths.

Remember B.E.N.D. when you evaluate your breathing. Just remind yourself a couple times a day, don't be militant about it. You have plenty of time to get better!

How can people tell if they're doing enough exercise or exercising intensely enough?

It all depends on your goals. Crossfitters are generally working out to destroy themselves. If you're just looking to get more active, any time you can work up a sweat is good. If you feel sluggish or have trouble focusing, I would suggest working out a little harder.

The way I see it is that most people don't exercise hard enough to accomplish the goals they have set for themselves. If you want to lose a lot of weight and look really good, running marathons probably isn't the best way to do it. For those looking to lose fat, lifting heavy weights is a low-impact way to exercise that sparks the hormone response you want.

How important is flexibility, when it comes to getting in shape? Why is this important?

Flexibility is touchy. Some need more of it, while some could use less of it. Yes, I said less.

Those people who don't move around a lot would benefit from a warm up that really focuses on increasing flexibility. The stereotypical person I think of is the middle aged guy who "doesn't have time for that girly stuff." Without flexibility, these people aren't training to their full potential. Plus, trying to force into a position they don't have the flexibility to reach causes detrimental movement compensations.

Then there are those who move entirely too much and need to learn to control their movements. The stereotypical person who fits in this category is the woman who loves group exercise classes. These people need more strength and control than they need flexibility. A lot of women have skewed perceptions of how flexible they are supposed to be. They stretch and stretch and stretch so that they can touch their palms on the floor like their gymnast friends, when in reality a toe touch of fingers to toes is normal.

Do minors typically need to get the permission of an adult or guardian, if they want to work with a personal trainer? If so, how does this work?

Generally the parent/guardian is the one paying. In these cases, an initial assessment is crucial. The parents of the athletes I have worked with have shown me that they just want to be sure their money is being put to good use. As a trainer, I'll explain my assessment and program design to the concerned (sometimes overbearing) parent, illustrating where their child is now, how far he or she has come, and where I plan to go next.

How will a trainer know what program is right for their client?

A few movement, position, and joint range of motion tests are key for me. This tells me what my client can or cannot do so that I can come up with a program that might fit them. I can restore them to a "normal" defined by the literature in terms of position and flexibility. Then I will modify the program if any more red flags come up when we work together. It's a constant game of trial and error, but the initial assessment keeps me from blindly guessing in my program design.

For people who are always tired, won't working out make them feel like they have even less energy?

Working out has never made me feel like I have less energy.

As you place exercise demands on your body, it gets used to mobilizing energy. Those physiologic pathways are then warmed up just like your oven is before you put dinner in it. Your appetite gets stabilized, and even though you eat more, you don't hold onto as much. The body's ability to adapt is remarkable.

What are the benefits of hiring a personal trainer over just buying some DVDs that feature personal trainers?

Coaching, coaching, and coaching. This is my biggest gripe with exercise books and DVDs. They don't put eyes on you. They can't make adjustments on the fly. And on that note, the program is set in stone. They don't have an initial assessment that tells them what things you should avoid or what things you need to focus on. Your exercise will not be tailored to your individual nature.

How much of a say should the client have in determining which exercises they do?

I can't give a percentage of how much say my client has, but I can tell you I listen to every request. If it's something they truly enjoy, even though I don't like the exercise for them, I'll likely let them do it. Ultimately, if your client isn't having fun, I'm not doing my job and they will leave me. And if they leave me, I can't help them at all.

Sometimes we actually want the same goal, but they aren't privy to the correct way to go about it. For example, I just wrote a program for a lady who wants to strengthen her neck with neck exercises. Neck exercises will do more harm than good because I know she's got a stiff neck secondary to an unstable and immobile torso. So what I will explain to her is that we're going to strengthen her neck by fixing the base that it sits on. I think this is the right way to go about things. If a client just wants me to program what they want to do, then what are they even paying me for?

Is it a good idea for someone to workout if they have a cold?

I would never try to push the intensity when you have a cold. If you have the ability to eat and the energy to exercise, I suggest some low intensity exercise to get the blood flowing. If you don't have the energy, however, don't feel bad. It's time to let your body recover.

Is it better to perform cardio before or after lifting weights or should cardio be done on a completely different day?

If you're looking to get bigger, the molecular pathways involved in building muscle are direct antagonists of traditional cardio. I would suggest this person avoid traditional cardio entirely and stick to high intensity activities.

Athletes need a more detailed schedule than I can prescribe here. Other general fitness clients may find cardio beneficial to their goals. For these people, I would suggest lifting weights before the cardio because it places higher demands on the central nervous system (CNS). You want the CNS fresh when try to pick up something heavy.

When people first start exercising, why do they sometimes gain weight initially?

As you start exercising, it's as if your body is experiencing an earthquake. A startled body basically says, "Well, if I'm going to have to start doing that from now on, I'm going to need more supplies."

This is where it starts to signal the growth of muscle, which is a storage site for things like the sugar you turn into energy. Without this initial weight gain, your body would not be able to progress as fast as it does.

If someone has a job where they don't move around a lot, what can they do to increase their activity during the day, when they're not working out?

If you work from home, play with a soccer ball during your work break. 10 minutes every hour or so helps me stay energized and focused on my job.

If you don't have the luxury of breaks, try out a standing desk. This is great if you can switch back and forth from seated to standing. If you can't move your work space up a level, kneel down on one or two knees at your desk. This is way more difficult than standing. Give it a shot!

If you need something more intense, hold a squat just above your seat. You can even do the same with a lunge, but I find it gets harder and harder to focus on work when you do this. Shoot for at least reps of 15 seconds and increase from there.

Trying to actually get a workout in when I'm stuck at the office never works for me. If you're the same way, the best plan is to go to the gym, even if for a short while, work really hard, and go home to recover. The harder your train, the more you get out of less time there.

HOW TO CONTACT US

Lance Goyke

Personal Trainer/Strength Coach for both

Indianapolis Fitness and Sports Training

&

LanceGoyke.com

Website: http://www.LanceGoyke.com

Email: lance@lancegoyke.com

INTERVIEW WITH TERRY BARGA

5 TRAINING LIKE A PROFESSIONAL

Life Fitness Academy is a holistic group of personal trainers, nutrition specialists, and fitness coaches. We believe that nutrition plays a vital role along with your fitness. We want the opportunity to show you how it has influenced us and how we can impact our community. We at Life Fitness Academy believe that our body, mind, spirit are all parts of our wellbeing. We believe whole health is a journey that should focus on every area of your life: spiritual, physical, and psychological. We have been where you are and love helping people out of that place and into whole health.

Why do people say, "Breakfast is the most important meal of the day"? Is there any truth in this?

When you eat isn't as important as what you eat. If your choices are to eat a donut or don't eat breakfast, don't eat breakfast. Eating something like that will take up to 48 hours to digest and because it takes so much energy to digest, it can leave you feeling more tired than if you skipped it. Concentrate more on giving your body the proper fuel to have energy for your day.

How can someone do resistance training if they don't own weights or belong to a gym?

You can easily use resistance bands in your home. You can find bands at most sporting goods stores and you can loop it around things in the room and do a variety of exercises. You have less chance of injuring yourself using a resistance band without supervision than with weights. Almost any moves with weights can be done with a resistance band.

Is it true that stress makes people gain weight? What is the truth, if any, behind this?

Cortisol is known as the stress hormone and is produced by the adrenal gland when you are stressed. It helps to support normal glucose metabolism, blood pressure levels, insulin release, immune function and inflammation levels, which means it can have some positive effects. When it's released in small amounts, cortisol can help you quickly tap into energy, memory, immunity, equilibrium and lower your sensitivity to pain.

When you're under chronic stress, however, increased levels of cortisol can wreak havoc by adversely affecting your brain, thyroid, blood sugar, bones, muscles, blood pressure, immunity and inflammation levels. Too much cortisol in the body, for instance, can result in foggy thinking, feeling run down, altered blood sugar levels and muscle discomfort. Cortisol can also affect your appetite.

Do personal trainers normally work with clients who are only free on weekends or during off-hours? What's typical in terms of when personal trainers are available?

Not at all. Unfortunately, many people have 9-5 jobs so the only time they can work out is early in the morning or in the evening. So it may be harder to schedule because those times are more in demand. Personally, as a full-time trainer, I would love more normal work hour appointments.

If someone has back problems, or other physical limitations, how can they lift weights safely, without getting hurt?

There are many other ways of working out without using weights. You need to heal and strengthen the injury or problem area before moving on to more challenging activities. This is where a trainer comes in handy, because they will know many ways to strengthen a muscle and they should also know your limits almost better than the client.

How should someone determine how many grams of protein and carbs they should be eating each day?

Well, textbook answer is 1.2-1.8 grams of protein per kilogram of body weight. 1 kg= 2.2lbs. Which turns out to not be as much as you think, a 6 oz. steak usually satisfies those numbers. It's not so important to worry about the specific amount as the kind of protein you are getting. Overdoing it can stress the adrenal glands, which can produce the stress hormone cortisol and actually sabotage your success.

You don't need a low-quality soy protein shake after your workout. Dark leafy greens have protein, certain grains like quinoa have protein as well. Then, of course, there are your meat, eggs, dairy, and nuts that are high in protein as well. Most people get enough from their diet. You want to get most of your carbs from vegetables and fruits.

You should avoid refined and processed grains and sugar like the plague. Think about what you're eating. Ask yourself, "how is this food going to help my body?" if you don't know, or know it won't help, walk away.

The new fad seems to be "buying organic". Is there any validity to eating organic food over non-organic food? What are the benefits and/or things to be aware of?

Conventional farming uses pesticides and genetically modified organisms. So buying organic you can at least avoid them. However like anything, there are pitfalls. We encourage you to know your local farmer and know how he produces your food. Then you have fresh, local, and likely organic foods.

The USDA must inspect a farm and the farmer must pay them, so many use organic methods, but don't get the USDA seal because of the cost. And then there are some certified organic farmers that probably cut corners. Know your farmer and eat time tested foods!

If someone reaches their fitness goals, should they still continue to work with a personal trainer?

That will depend on the person. Once you reach your goals, you will still need to do something to maintain your fitness level and expend some energy. If you can do that on your own, then maybe it's not necessary to keep a trainer. If, however, you need someone to tell you what to do and push you and keep you accountable, maybe keep meeting with your trainer once a week or so.

Hopefully your trainer has given you an education to take with you so you won't be dependent on them for the rest of your life. Find a trainer/teacher and learn.

Most experts seem to all agree that nuts are very healthy, but they seem to have a lot of fat in them. Won't eating high fat foods like nuts make it more difficult to lose weight?

Absolutely not. Its SUGAR & things that your body processes as sugar that make you gain weight, not fat. Fat is the body's preferred method of energy. You need to replace bad, stored fat with good fats like nuts and avocados. In addition, vitamins A,D,E and K (found in a lot of green veggies) are fat soluble which means they NEED fats to be transported throughout your body. Often times when you see foods that are low fat, they have removed some fat and replaced it with sugar, or worse, artificial sweeteners.

How important is nutrition if someone works out consistently?

Nutrition is extremely important. When you eat better, you will feel better in your workout. So in order to keep your workouts at their peak, you should eat the best you can. Once you've reached your goals, it is much easier to maintain without working out as much when you eat the way you should. We often say nutrition is 80% of the problem.

Why do people have such a hard time losing belly fat?

Belly fat is totally related to nutrition. Too much sugar, refined carbs, sodas and alcohol are usually the culprits of belly fat. You must cut out white flour and sugar to get rid of belly fat.

HOW TO CONTACT US
Terry Barga
Owner/Operator of Life Fitness Academy
Phone: 615-562-2633
Email: lifefitnessacademy@gmail.com

INTERVIEW WITH DERRICK SOBOTKA

6 GETTING A HELPING HAND

Since 1998, Barry's Bootcamp has been delivering "The Best Workout in the World" to a legendary following, including many celebrities. Our no-nonsense, results driven reputation may intimidate some newcomers, but they quickly discover that Barry's Bootcamp delivers an affordable, efficient and fun workout in a night club party environment that is nothing like the cliche boot camps found in every town.

What are some of the most common myths about nutrition?

I think the most common myth about nutrition is that it doesn't matter. In actuality your results are 60% in the kitchen. Without a positive relationship with food the workout is always going to suffer.

I like to describe the difference between a "diet" and "your diet" as two very different things. A "diet" is never going to work...it is a temporary fix for a long term issue. "Your diet" is your relationship with food. How often do you eat? What do you eat?

How does your relationship with food effect the results that you see from your workout. How do you need to change your relationship with food? Once you answer those questions and change the puzzle pieces that don't fit then you are on the road to a successful body.

What is a "drop set"?

A drop set is a commonly used term in exercise when you are attempting to reach total and complete failure in a specific muscle group. Let's take for example a bicep curl. You performing a bicep curl with a twenty pound set of weights to failure. When you reach that point of failure where you cannot perform another repetition you immediately drop down to a lower weight and continue that bicep curl. The philosophy is to take the specific muscle group to a point at which you might never have before.

If someone has a friend who is in good shape, who is willing to give them exercise advice, why is it still a good idea to hire a personal trainer?

There is no denying that a friend who is in good shape might know some great tips about exercising. A personal trainer, however, is educated and specialized in the finer things regarding exercise. Safety, perfect form, physical limitations and responsible exercise program design are all areas where a personal trainer is a master of. A personal trainer has the materials and know-how to track your progress. Education is power.

What are some tips to help people stick with an exercise program and not quit?

I have my clients do something a bit unorthodox to stay on track with their exercise program. I have my clients find a bathing suit, pair of skinny jeans, a dress, anything that they aspire to be able to fit in to. I have them purchase this article of clothing and hang it in their home where they will see it every single day. I also have them try it on or attempt to try it on once a month. Their goal is to fit into this article of clothing.

Almost every single time the client finally gets to the point to where they fit into this article of clothing. They met their goal!!! Sometimes that article of clothing ends up being too small!!! We have to celebrate our wins in life and seeing physical progress is always the most motivational.

How can people overcome junk food cravings?

I think that everyone struggles with cravings. We all have our little favorite snacks that we know we shouldn't have. It feels bad and sometimes feeling bad feels so good! I tend to have a fairly controversial way of doing things so what do I suggest? HAVE IT! Have a bite.

If you are craving cookies...have a bite. But just one bite. You would be shocked that just with one bite your craving will completely go away and then finish that hunger off with a positive food choice. Have a bite of that cookie and then move on to having a piece of fruit.

You are craving that cookie because your body is wanting something sweet. Give it what it wants...have the bite of the cookie and finish off that sweet tooth with the natural sugars from the fruit. Your body really doesn't know the difference. We have to trick it.

How does someone know if they're "over-training"?

There is a fine line between soreness due to training and soreness due to over training. Feeling a little bit sore from training is a perfectly normal feeling to have. Especially if you haven't exercised in a long time. Now if that soreness does not go away in a day or two you are over training. You shouldn't "hurt" from training you should feel the muscle responding to the stress you just put it under.

How does someone tone up and lose fat under their arms and around their triceps?

Interval cardiovascular work is always an important element of any workout program. It is very difficult, almost impossible, to just "spot treat" a specific problem area. The fat burning element of interval cardio is essential to reducing the fat from the problem areas. From that point you want to dive into resistance training.

If you want to tone up your arms you would transition into resistance training. Building lean muscle in any area is going to burn fat more efficiently when coupling it with your interval cardiovascular work. In the case of the arms. Always integrate the interval cardiovascular work to reduce the fat stores and then work with some isolated tricep work with movements like a tricep kickback, tricep pull-down, or an overhead tricep press.

What's the difference between "good carbs" and "bad carbs"?

There are carbs in almost anything you eat to a certain degree. The question is "what are they and what are they doing for you?" A bad carb is a carbohydrate that is or is made up of highly processed foods. These carbs will drastically spike your blood sugar.

You will also never really feel satisfied. You need some carbs for energy though. So how do we get them? Unrefined food. Take whole grains, vegetables, fruits or beans. All of these foods have carbohydrates in them and yet they are unrefined foods. Our body can identify them and use them to their fullest potential. We can use them completely.

What should people look out for when hiring a personal trainer?

Don't be afraid to do your homework. A good personal trainer should have their credentials in order to present to you. Are they certified, and not only that, are they certified through a reputable certification program. Ask them! Ask to see their certification or credentials. Also...what do their current or former clients have to say?

Don't be afraid to ask for references. A good trainer should be able to provide you with personal testimonies from clients who have used their professional services. Ask them about their experiences. Do your homework when you are putting your health in another person's hands.

What are some of the most common misconceptions that people have about hiring a personal trainer?

I think the most common misconception that I hear about hiring a personal trainer is that it is way too expensive. I generally like to put it into perspective for them. A personal trainer can run you anywhere from $75 per hour session all the way up to sometimes $200 per session. Even on the highest end of that pay scale a heart attack will cost you on average, including medication and doctor visits, roughly $50,000.00 per year for the rest of your life. I personally would much rather prevent that expense all together and pay the $75.00 to $200.00 as an investment toward my health.

HOW TO CONTACT US
Derrick Sobotka

Manager / Trainer Barry's Bootcamp

Website: www.barrysbootcamp.com

Phone: (619) 906-4455

Email: derrick@barrysbootcamp.com

INTERVIEW WITH IRV RUBENSTEIN

7 GETTING THE JOB DONE

Steps was founded in 1986 by myself and a fellow grad student in exercise science at Peabody College of Vanderbilt University, Nashville, TN. Our Intent was to introduce Nashville to a personal training facility where fitness professionals could rent time and space to provide their services to their own clients. In 1989 we opened our first facility and moved into our current location in 2000. Today about 20 trainers ply their trade as either independent operators (their own clientele) or independent contractors (training steps-derived clients).

What are the best foods that people should eat to gain energy and why are these foods so important?

Carbohydrates are the body's preferred source of energy with simpler versions most accessible shortly before and immediately after an exercise event/session and complex carbs for longer term energy storage and replenishment. For longer term exercise, fats are necessary; healthier fats are preferred, such as nuts and vegetable oils.

Is it better to lift weights with free weights or with weight machines? Why is one better than the other?

There are two ways to approach this question: For whom, and why? Without going into a dissertation on it, suffice it to say that there are times, clients, and exercises where machines are better or more apropos than free weights. While the latter are 'better' in that they more closely approximate the way our bodies have to actually stabilize a joint or joints in order to move another or others, and they do allow more 'functional' movement patterns overall, machines do serve a purpose.

For one, of all the major exercises – the pull from a high position – few people can do a pull up or chin up, so a lat pull will strengthen these most integral muscles for many sports and life activities – the forearm, biceps and lats. The other value to machines is for people who may require total stabilization and isolation at some phase of their training in order to strengthen muscles that will contribute to more functional movements.

Thus, for generally older clients with osteoarthritis of the knees or hips, machines allow one to condition muscles of the lower extremities without contributing to the already-worn out joints that would otherwise need to be done in closed-chain moves such as squats and lunges. For these and several other reasons I refuse to elevate one modality over another.

If someone needs to quickly lose a few pounds for a special occasion, what's the best way they can do this?

Cut calories. For the most part, Americans overeat as much as 25-50% of their caloric needs. I recommend cutting one-third of their total caloric intake from all their preferred food choices, even desserts. Doing so allows them to eat as they wish but cut calories in the process. If one has to cut more calories to lose weight prior to a special occasion, they could shift their macronutrient composition toward more proteins – but they need to drink more water to prevent the metabolic downsides from diminishing their energy and the effects of Ketosis that accompanies high protein diets.

What types of shoes should people wear when working out?

It depends on what kind of workout. If relatively static but needing support/cushioning, a cross trainer or even a low cost pair of K-Mart shoes will suffice. If you will be doing movements such as agility or plyometrics, you may need a different shoe to accommodate the surface, type of moves, and speeds at which you're doing them.

Can someone use a personal trainer to help them rehabilitate from a sports injury? How would this be handled?

Yes. But I would suggest one seeks a trainer with a more advanced education or more years of experience. Getting a referral from a doctor or therapist will provide some assurance of qualifications and understanding of the nature of the problem and a hint of experience with other clients who'd seen him/her.

Is it possible to lose fat and gain muscle at the same time? If so, how can this be done effectively?

Clearly this is more possible for males, and for younger people than older people. Studies do not show that middle age women can readily build muscle – 1-2# is what many short-term studies show. (Few studies of this nature have gone beyond 6 months so it's hard to say what those numbers look like.) Losing fat is best accomplished by cutting calories, plus cardio exercise at moderate or high intensities.

Adding large body movement exercises such as squats, lunges, chest presses, overhead presses, pull downs and rows, plus many of the 'fuctional' and Olympic exercises, ensures greater caloric burn plus greater muscle accretion if, and I do mean if, the resistances are high enough to generate protein accretion. Many older folks are not willing to work that hard but if they do, they can build some muscle. It helps to be male, however.

How soon, after someone starts a diet and exercise program, should they start to see results, to know if their diet and exercise program is working?

It's a matter of what results one is trying to achieve. If we're talking weight loss or size loss, it could be 4-8 weeks before those results show up. If it's strength or function, it could be within 2-4 weeks. If it's definition or hypertrophy, it could be 8-16 weeks. But if it's to feel and move better, it could be almost immediately. Some people simply need to start moving more to feel better.

If someone is a heavy smoker, should their workout routine be adjusted at all? If so, how?

It depends on age and other health factors. Young heavy smokers, while at greater risk than non-smokers of similar activity status – presumably sedentary – can be pushed pretty hard, almost as hard as a previously sedentary person. Older heavy smokers are likely to have co-morbidities such as hypertension, heart disease, etc. and should be regarded from that perspective rather than just their smoking habit.

Is there any truth to the claim that exercise can help improve brain function and/or mental focus? If yes, how?

Yes, definitely. Several studies published in 2012 have demonstrated improved cognitive function and memory in those who do regular cardio exercise; some second-half of 2012 have shown similar though lesser benefits from resistance training programs. Those few that have combined the two modalities have shown benefits closer to those of cardio-only programs.

As to how these occur, the first thoughts have to do with blood flow overall but obviously to the brain. Secondary mechanisms are hypothesized to come through neurological relationships with the musculoskeletal movements that all forms of exercise demand. In fact, these may be more a factor for benefits from a resistance training program as the moves are more diverse, multi-directional, multi-factorial – Think balance and stability both of specific joints as well as the body itself – and usually more demanding – think intensity at the end of a set of series of sets, which requires mental input. There are probably some hormonal and metabolic inputs to the benefits of exercise, from insulin levels to blood sugar control, too.

Can couples or groups of people workout with a personal trainer at the same time?

Of course. Is it possible to be as observant of new clients especially while teaching or performing more complex moves? If treated properly, and taught progressively, yes, although many instructors fail to take into consideration the variety of limitations and needs of all the participants in a class format. Thus, If one's needs are greater, the smaller the group, the better for the client.

HOW TO CONTACT US
Irv Rubenstein
President/CEO of STEPS, Inc.
Phone: 615- 269-8855
Email: irvrube@gmail.com

INTERVIEW WITH GREGG SCHWARTZ

8 EATING YOUR WAY TO A HEALTHIER BODY

American Mobile Fitness is an innovative company. Our mission is to offer a comfortable place for people to workout, to design challenging and customized routines, to motivate and encourage clients to reach their goals, and to get people the results they desire through personal training, group exercise and group training. We provide convenient personal training, group exercise, and group training in our clients' homes or offices. We bring all the equipment you need for a great workout. You may also come to our state of the art studio and get the results you want. Our goal is to make fitness more convenient. We want to help you achieve a healthy lifestyle while maintaining a busy schedule. Our clients don't have to worry about time constraints. We make ourselves available at their convenience.

What can thin people do to build muscle?

The key to building muscle is to lift weights and eat a high protein diet. You should pick a weight that you can only lift 6-8 reps and do 3 -5 sets when you are looking to build muscle. Thin statured individuals are limited on how big they can get based on their build. Genetics sometimes holds us back and you can only build yourself as big as your frame will allow.

What are some factors that impact people's metabolism?

Metabolism is a measurement of what your body is burning off. As a person ages their metabolism decreases. As people are more or less active their metabolism will increase or decrease. Just living we burn off so many calories. This can be measured for each individual through a device called a MedGem which measures your carbon dioxide output. When we are more active and workout we will increase our metabolism. When we build muscle on our bodies we will also increase metabolism and turn our bodies into a furnace. This is because our bodies have to maintain the new muscle which requires more energy to survive and in turn increases metabolism. Yo- yo dieting and quick or excessive weight loss will decrease metabolism due to the loss of muscle.

What can people do to stay motivated, after they've started a workout program?

Once you start a workout program it is important to set realistic goals. Always try to workout with a friend that is at the same level as you to keep you going. Always change your program or routine so you don't hit a plateau. You have to remember never to watch the scale. Our weight changes all the time and it is not about weight it is truly about inches and percentage of body fat for a better looking body.

Can sit-ups help people lose belly fat? Why do some people do thousands of sit-ups and they still don't lose any belly fat?

Our bodies do not have the capability to spot reduce. When you do sit ups you are able to increase the strength of the abdominals and also the core. The key to losing fat around the midsection is to eat clean and lose overall percent body fat. Genetics also plays a roll and some people no matter how hard they try will never be able to get that six pack abs.

If someone has a personal trainer, do they also need a nutritionist? What are the differences between a personal trainer and a nutritionist?

A personal trainer specializes in exercise and designing specific programs to get people the best results based on their ability level. A nutritionist specializes in food and healthy eating programs for special populations. Depending on how in depth you want to be you could have both. Many personal trainers do have nutrition backgrounds. They can give you an idea of how much carbohydrates, proteins, and fats you should have in your diet. Depending on the state it is determined how much nutritional information a personal trainer can give you. A nutritionist does have some knowledge of exercise but cannot develop a specific program.

What is "core strength"?

The core is comprised of your back abdominals and your lumbo pelvic hip complex. Every movement our bodies make your core subconsciously contracts seconds before the movement is made. Your core is the foundation of all movements in your body. Everyone needs core strength to be able to make efficient movements without injuries. Yours limbs will only be as strong as your core. If you have a weak core it will be hard for your body to function correctly. Core strength is one of the most important aspects of fitness.

Why is it better to eat more frequent, smaller meals throughout the day than less frequent larger meals?

It is important to eat small frequent meals preferably every 2 hours. This is important to keep your metabolism going. It is a lot easier for your body to digest smaller meals. When people eat less frequently they tend to overeat. People that snack throughout the day tend to keep their weight in the recommend range and stay in good shape.

How often should someone workout with a personal trainer?

A person should strength train 2-3 times per week. It is important to have a trainer vary the routine so you can maximize your results.

Every day, there seems to be a new "health food" product on the grocery store shelves. How can people tell if a food item is really healthy or not?

When it comes to health foods and supplements you have to be careful. Consumers have to remember that supplements are not regulated. Whatever it says on the label does not have to be in the product. Look at the label. Food should have no more than 5 ingredients. If it has more than that do not buy it. Many diet foods are full of fillers that are not good. There are third party companies that help regulate products. Look for their inspection labels. The best thing to purchase is whole foods. Do not buy anything processed.

What is a healthy amount of weight to lose each week? Why is it a bad idea to lose more weight than this each week?

One pound a week is ideal for weight loss. Losing more weight to quickly will actually cause the body to stop losing weight. Our bodies have safety mechanisms and if you lose weight to quickly it will store more fat and burn up your muscle. In turn it will decrease your metabolism and you will gain weight. As we lose weight we lose twice as much muscle as we do fat. It is important to strength train as you lose weight.

What happens at the initial appointment with a personal trainer?

Trainers should do a full fitness assessment at the initial appointment with a new client. It is important to establish a baseline of where the client is at so you know how to progress them and get them results. It is important to go over resting heart rate, target heart rate zone, blood pressure, strength testing, cardiovascular testing, flexibility testing, percentage of body fat, circumference measurements, and a full medical history that includes any medications and supplements the client may be on.

There seems to be a lot of talk about these "cleansing diets", where people just drink lemon juice with cayenne pepper and some sort of syrup for 30 or more days. Is this safe and/or healthy? Why or why not?

Cleansing diets are worse than fad diets. Diets are a bad word and cannot be sustained over a long period of time and in turn people gain weight back. It is important to learn how to eat so it can be sustained over long periods. It is not safe for your body to lose too much weight too quickly. If it does it is so easy to put it all back on. Most of these cleansing diets are basically starving the body and have no nutritional value. If is important to just eat frequent healthy meals throughout the day. Exercise daily and you will get the results you are looking for.

HOW TO CONTACT US

Gregg Schwartz

Owner / Personal Trainer at American Mobile Fitness

Website: www.AmericanMobileFitness.com

Phone: 419-351-1381

Email: info@AmericanMobileFitness.com

INTERVIEW WITH JAY SIEFERT

9 TIPS TO PICK THE BEST WORKOUT PROGRAM

Studio Element Personal Training is a private, intimate fitness training facility in St. Louis that offers healthy & effective solutions to weight loss, sport-specific training, nutritional counseling, strength building & flexibility. We tailor our fitness programs to the goals, abilities, and limits of our clients.

What are "boot camps" and why are they so popular?

Boot camps are usually a high intensity group workout that takes place in a gym, outdoors, or even in a facility like a gymnastics center. They have gained popularity in recent years for a couple of reasons. The group, peer support dynamic appeals to many who have had struggles on their own. Also, boot camp style programs are typically offered at an affordable price.

Are there ways to reduce recovery time or soreness between workouts, without taking supplements?

Most importantly, proper rest is an essential component to any fitness program. With so many high intensity workout programs now available, our industry is seeing a fair share of overuse injuries. Beyond rest, a thorough stretching program and foam rolling are ways to reduce tightness and muscle soreness.

Fish seems to have a lot of fat in it. Will people gain weight if they eat too much fish?

As with any food item, eating too much of one thing could always have a potential for negative side effects. With that said, fish contains the type of fat called Omega 3's which have been shown to lower triglyceride levels. I would recommend including fish in your diet 2-3 times per week. Will someone gain weight if they eat too much fish? Most people, unless they have a metabolism disorder, will gain weight if the eat too much of anything.

What can people do to avoid back injuries when they're lifting weights?

We commonly see clients come into Studio Element with back issues. Preventative care is what tends to have the most impact on future back issues. Building a solid core, coupled with an all around well balanced fitness regimen can help support the back during resistance training. Proper form is also a key with any exercise involving the back. Enlisting the assistance of a qualified personal trainer will pay off greatly.

When is a spotter needed for exercises?

A spotter is needed for any exercise where there is a significant amount of effort being performed. Anytime someone is pushing their boundaries and/or trying a new, heavier weight, it is always smart to have a spotter close by.

How many grams of fat should people consume each day, if they want to lose weight?

There are many variables that must be taken into the equation of how much fat, protein, and anything else that should be ingested each day. These variables include body size, amount of weight to lose, activity level, and age. Also, what works for one person, does not work for another. The best scenario would be to consult with a Registered Dietician to develop a plan that specifically addresses your uniqueness.

How much sleep should people get when they exercise regularly?

Regular exercisers should ideally get 8-9 hours of sleep per night. As I mentioned earlier, rest is a vital component of any fitness program. In order to heal and grow properly, adequate and consistent rest is very necessary.

Is there any truth to the claim that exercise can help improve brain function and/or mental focus? If yes, how?

Physical exercise has been proven to improve brain function by increasing circulation and memory. It also increases blood flow to the brains leading to a more efficient delivery of oxygen and glucose and the removal of waste products.

Why do certain "non-fat" foods still make people gain weight?

People tend to eat quite a bit more when they know that a food item is non-fat, partially because these foods don't satisfy hunger like a full fat item does.

What is the difference between a "high impact" and a "low impact" workout?

A high impact workout is a workout where there is some kind of physical impact on the body. Many plyometric exercises, where you leave the ground, have the element of impact. More grounded, or closed-chain movements tend to be low to no impact. These are exercises where you don't leave the ground.

What is the typical way to pay a personal trainer? Weekly? Monthly? At each session?

There are several ways that you can pay for personal training sessions. Some facilities have monthly options, some have 3 or 6 month commitments, and some have pay up front in bulk options. Typically, the longer term that you commit to or the more you purchase upfront, the more affordable the price is per session.

I would always recommend spending a great deal of time researching the qualifications of any trainer. It would be much more desirable to pay a little more for someone who will efficiently get you the results you desire without injury.

Some opt to take the cheaper option of a trainer who has little in terms of qualifications and end up getting injured and achieve little in terms of results.

Should people with low blood sugar do anything differently before, during, or after a workout?

People with low blood sugar should definitely take some precaution with exercise. It would be smart to eat some kind of fast acting carb prior to exercise like fruit, oatmeal, or a banana. Having some type of fruit juice or even candy is recommended to have with you during your workouts if you run into an issue.

HOW TO CONTACT US
Jay Siefert
President of Studio Element
Website: www.studio-element.net
Email: jaysiefert@studio-element.net

UNITED PRINT PUBLISHERS

INTERVIEW WITH STEVE & TORI BRADFORD

10 A CERTAIN WAY DOES HELP

Center-Fit was founded by two personal trainers, a husband and wife team, Steve & Tori Bradford. We now have turned our goal focused personal training into small group exercise classes including kettlebells, boxing, yoga, zumba, and bootcamps.

Is it true that it's bad to eat too much fruit because of all of the sugar it contains?

While fruit does contain a lot of sugar grams technically, the sugar comes from a natural and unprocessed source (fructose). We believe that the healthiest foods you can eat come from the ground and were made by God and not man.

So no, fruit is not "bad" because of the sugar, however the quantity is important. For example, I wouldn't sit down to eat 4 bananas at once, but 1 banana while high in sugar is perfectly suitable and even nourishing to the body.

Is it true that exercise and a healthy diet can help reduce the chance of developing diabetes? If this is true, how can exercise and/or a good nutrition plan help prevent diabetes?

Yes it is true that nourishing nutrition and purposeful movement can help prevent the risk of developing Type 2 Diabetes. Diabetes is a disease based on the body's inability to efficiently utilize blood sugar and recognize insulin. It has been proven that the types of foods we eat affect our blood sugars because of the speed at which the food is broken down. Foods are considered to be "high-glycemic" when the blood sugar spikes after the food has been ingested. These foods are normally carbohydrates that have been highly processed and refined so the body breaks them down quickly. The more often these foods are eaten, the body becomes bogged down with these high levels of blood sugars and it can cause problems for the pancreas creating an insensitivity to the body's insulin thus creating the onset of diabetes. Exercise also plays a role in managing blood sugar because muscles use blood sugar as energy, so if a person does not purposefully move like in exercise the body does not use energy a.k.a. blood sugar. Purposeful movement creates an environment for the muscles to call on blood sugar to be used as energy, thus using any extra blood sugar that the body may have in the blood stream.

What's the difference between "aerobic" and "anaerobic" exercises?

It's the difference between a marathon runner and a sprinter. A marathon runner, similar to aerobic exercise, uses long steady oxygen, where as anaerobic exercise like the sprinter uses quick bursts of energy/oxygen and would be unable to sustain that level of intensity for a long period of time.

Are certain types of cardio workouts better than others?

Yes absolutely! A lot of research points to interval trainings being a much more efficient form of cardio workouts that maximizes total caloric burn, as well as burns a higher percentage of those calories coming from fat.

Who should the average person talk to about which exercise program would be best for them?

We recommend speaking with someone that has certifications in the area they are training in from a reputable organization. The fitness industry is full of trainers that only took a test online and may or may not have any real experience with movement patterns or health. Anyone can give you a good workout that burns calories, but a true trainer will have knowledge on how the body SHOULD move and why.

Does a person have to check with their doctor before beginning a workout program with a personal trainer?

It is always recommended that a person check with their regular physician before beginning any new exercise program. While exercise and purposeful movement is great for the body, many people need to take it slow at the beginning.

Is it a good idea to workout when feeling mentally stressed? Why or why not?

Purposeful movement in the form of a workout routine can be extremely beneficial for reducing mental and emotional stress. There are many reasons for this including the increase in endorphins that are released, the feeling of accomplishment, and of course achieving goals. I believe the main reason for this is called meditation in movement which is the concept that while you are focusing on the movement or exercise at hand, you are no longer focusing on the stresses of your day or life, therefore reducing any stress that you may have been dealing with before you started your workout.

In addition to working out, what are some of the most beneficial activities to participate in and why are these activities so beneficial/healthy?

We recommend that everyone live an active lifestyle. It's great to have a regular workout routine, but the most important aspect of a healthy life is consistency in movement. These activities can include the whole family and should be fun like playing sports, hiking, biking, etc. Including these activities in your daily life will be beneficial for your family and their health.

How long should a personal training session last?

Most personal training sessions last either 30 minutes or 60 minutes. We utilize hard style kettle bells in most of our training sessions which are very efficient tools and workouts can be completed in less time with the same caloric and fat burn as in traditional workouts.

How do people get rid of loose skin after weight loss?

Well the only natural way to get rid of loose skin is to lose the weight slow and steady so that the body has time to adapt to this loss in fat. The younger a person is the easier this process is because the elasticity of the skin is still very strong, as a person ages they begin to lose this elasticity.

What are some tips that people should keep in mind, for practicing good form during their workouts?

We are big advocates of maintaining good form in their workouts, not just because their workout will be more efficient, but because they will reduce the risk of overuse injuries to their joints and tendons. Some good tips would include not doing something if it hurts, workout barefoot so you can feel the ground on all four corners of your feet, keep the knees over the ankles, hips over knees, shoulders over hips, and chin up.

Do people have to join the gym that their personal trainer belongs to, in order to hire them?

This policy changes with each gym, so you should check with your trainer. Many trainers are available to train in your home, or even in a small studio. In my experience, the best trainers have their own studios or work for themselves, so you should seek them out in your area.

HOW TO CONTACT US

Steve & Tori Bradford

Owners, Personal and Group Trainers of Center-Fit

Website: center-fit.com

Phone: 630-449-7331

Email: info@center-fit.com

CONCLUSION

Congratulations on making it to the end of this book! We hope that you realize and appreciate the immense level of real world knowledge that you've just acquired. The one thing you may be feeling, at this point, is a bit of "information overload", due to the many tips, pieces of advice, and strategies that are jammed into this book. If you are feeling a bit overwhelmed from everything you've just learned, allow us to offer you one final piece of advice: Take a day to let your brain absorb all of the information you just learned. As they say: "Sleep on it". If you attempt to try and remember and implement everything you just learned, your efforts may tend to be scattered and a bit unorganized. Instead, take a day off from the information. If you do this, you're likely to find that you develop a sense of clarity and a better perspective on the information.

Once you've taken a day to allow yourself to re-focus in this way, we encourage you to slowly go back through the book, writing down the actionable information that you intend to implement. Simply reading and understanding the information is not enough. By writing down the information that you plan on implementing, it will allow you to put a clear plan of action into place for yourself.

As you go through the information, don't worry about the order in which you write things down. The first thing to do is to just get the information down on paper. There are many great strategies and tips within this book, but the goal here is for you to extract the exact advice that you will be taking action on. Don't worry if you are unsure about whether or not you will be taking immediate action on certain advice. Just write down everything that you may possibly take action on.

Once you've compiled this list of action steps and "maybe action steps", begin to prioritize this list. In other words, re-write the list with the actions that you know you're going to take at the top of the list and the action items that you may not take action on towards the bottom of the list. By organizing your list in this way, you will be able to build a practical, useable to-do list, from the information you learned in this book. Once you've done this, you will be in an excellent position to start taking focused steps, with clarity and purpose.

It is our hope that you, as the reader, will take real world action on the information you've learned here.

Wishing you all the best in your action-taking, fitness and nutrition endeavors!